BINAY'S STRATEGY
FOR OVERCOMING
AMBROSIA

BINAY'S STRATEGY
— FOR OVERCOMING —
AMBROSIA

DR BINAY SINGH

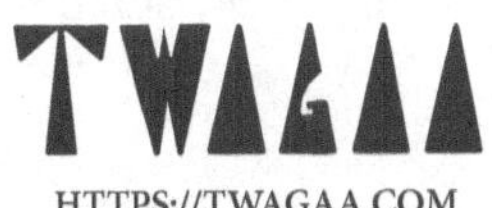

HTTPS://TWAGAA.COM

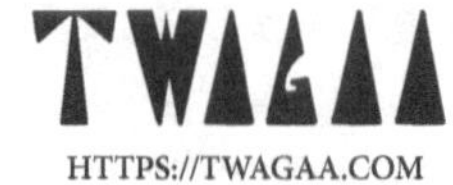

Mumbai (MH), India
Website: https://twagaa.com
Email: hello@twagaa.com

First published by TWAGAA INTERNATIONAL

Title: Binay's Strategy for Overcoming Ambrosia

ISBN: 978-93-92849-32-9

First Edition
Published in India

Ordering Information:
Quantity sales: Special discounts are available on quantity purchases by corporations, associations, and others. For details, contact the publisher at the address or email above.

ACKNOWLEDGEMENTS

I am very blessed that today my higher power praises me and pushes me to add value to others' lives, to make our Ukrainian people healthier. My focus is especially on the people of Odessa. Together, we can overcome any challenge that we face. Even something like ambrosia, which has persisted for such a long time, is no match for our combined efforts. This book is for you, my friends and neighbors.

CONTENTS

CHAPTER 1

THE TRUTH ABOUT AMBROSIA

For a very long time, people around the world have struggled to deal with their allergies. Peanut butter, pollen, antibiotics: there is a wide range of allergies, their effects ranging from the minor to the severe. Allergy symptoms can become particularly frustrating when they depend on a person's environment, though. When you are content with the place that you live in, happy with the landscape and the community, and yet it keeps you *sick* a large portion of the year, you may feel helpless, as if there is nothing that you can do to clear out your own space and find true satisfaction.

This is the experience that an ambrosia allergy entails.

The truth about ambrosia is that no matter how hard you try to manage it, you may still feel like you have made no progress whatsoever. You will look at all the other people around you, feeling happy and comfortable, only suffering through sniffles or congestion on the rare occasion that they fall ill, and you wonder, *Why me?* The pain is never unbearable, not *quite*. It would not seem so bad at all, if only there were some way to flip a switch. If you could choose to experience the symptoms for a moment and then turn them back off again, the way that you turn off a faucet or a light, then you could live with them.

Ambrosia would not seem so bad, if that were the case.

Ambrosia is not so kind as that, however. Its symptoms seep into all parts of your life, threatening to upend even the simplest of all your pleasures. It is relentless in its effects, torturing you when you wake up and never letting down, right up to the time that you lay your head on your pillow and make a bumpy descent into dreamland.

Have *you* experienced ambrosia allergy symptoms before?

The itchy, watery eyes are a giveaway. They become more and more discomfiting the longer they last. Like a puff of dust that you cannot quite shake, the itchiness seems to run deep. It starts out somewhere behind your retina and then bubbles up above your eyelid. If you rub your eyes, the feeling only gets worse. You realize that there is no relief from this itchiness. It is an itch that you cannot scratch, an incessant knocking at the door that you cannot answer.

As if that were not terrible enough, a scratchy throat follows. That is how the allergy works for many people: it will find a way down across your face. What seemed to impact only your eyes will then settle into your respiratory system. Every breath will take tremendous effort. You will feel as if something is constricting your airway. You try to breathe further down in your lungs, but to no avail. The tightness is inescapable. You wonder what you could have ever done to deserve a punishment like this. Without any sign or hint as to what is going on, your throat betrays you.

Of course, it makes a stop along the way. Before landing in your throat, the ambrosia allergy will hit your nasal passage too. A runny nose or congestion is another of the most common symptoms of ambrosia allergy. You run your arm across your nostril, coming away with a mess that you need to wash away. Try to wipe it up with some tissues, and as quickly as you have opened up a box, it is empty. There is no stemming the rush that your allergy incites. The ambrosia is ceaseless in the nastiness that it compels.

Coughing and wheezing will make your ambrosia allergy all the more conspicuous. If you had thought you would be able to at least keep your allergy a secret from all the people around you, you were wrong. Everyone will know immediately that you are going through *something*. They will hear it in the mad way that you hack up your mucus. It will become more painful as you tear up the back of your throat, creating tiny cuts so that each breath becomes a chore.

From there, you may incur sinus pressure, which may cause facial pain. This is one of the most awful symptoms of an ambrosia allergy. You will feel like your nose is going to collapse in on itself, like there is a heavy air following you around wherever you go. Go into a different office, and the air is there as well. It is wherever you are because the problem is not with the air per se – but the particles that are in the air. Filled with ambrosia, the air becomes like a toxin to you, causing you to feel all manners of things that you would never feel intentionally.

Swollen, bluish-colored skin beneath the eyes is another common, unpleasant symptom of an ambrosia allergy. Over and over, your friends and family will ask you if you have been getting enough sleep. While the answer will likely be *no* regardless, you know that the discoloration would persist all the same. With sleep or without it, your eyes would appear unhealthy, like someone has taken something out of you – an essence of your personality removed, your energy watered down and diluted. You will sense that if you had to take on a fresh challenge, you would *not* be able to show up and perform your best at it.

You look for any respite from all of these symptoms. None will come, though. A decreased sense of smell or taste tends to follow. What little joys you had, the peace that you found when you were eating your favorite meal or drinking your favorite beverage, they all disappear. There are no more small joys. Instead, you itch constantly. You think back longingly on how *delicious* your lunch could be. None of that does anything, though. None of your wishing and wanting will ever get you anywhere. It is a carrot dangling in front of your nose, with nothing but the stick to keep you trotting along.

Poor sleep quality will drive in all of these pains. When you are going on six hours, four hours, or even less sleep, you will wonder how life could *get* so uncomfortable. The ambrosia will rob you of your sense of self. Whereas you used to feel strong and capable, actualization will slip through your fingers. You will doubt all your own talents and skills because the lack of sleep will haunt you. It will terrorize you seven nights of the week, forcing you to take long naps on the weekends when you ought to be spending time with your friends and family.

This is an allergic condition. It is every bit as awful as it sounds. Anyone else who has overcome an ambrosia allergy can attest that this is true. If you are managing an ambrosia allergy yourself, then you are in the depths at this moment. You hear me talking about the symptoms, and it all feels like an *attack*.

That is not my intention, though. I do not want to attack you – but to help you. My goal is to show you how I have overcome my ambrosia allergy so that you can do the same. All of us can get to that point, to the relief that we long for.

If you are ready to take action, then I am ready to guide you. From there, your greatest life is within your reach. Before I explain what you should do, though, let me give you an overview of my *own* journey in this area.

CHAPTER 2

MY EXPERIENCE

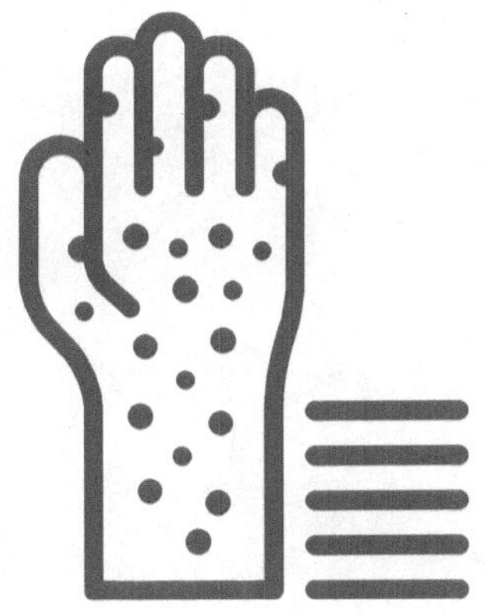

Many a night, I have sat up scratching at my eyes or coughing until my chest hurt. I would look over at the clock, as the hours ticked away. By the time half of my night passed, I knew that I would feel sick all of the next day. It would get to me, the lack of sleep. To know that it was a plant that was causing it, not anything that I was eating or taking but something in the air, felt like there was nothing I could do to help myself. The pain was not horrific, but it was never-ending. I knew that I had to do something. With bated breath, I would wait for the morning to arrive, hoping that it would do something to change my situation.

The daytime was, however, even more oppressive than the nighttime. When the sun was out, I would remember all the times when I had felt so much better. They would come rushing back to me, to torment me with reminiscences of a clear throat and eyes at ease. There was a lure to them, which made the allergy symptoms even *worse*. I felt the better times pulling me toward them. Still, nothing could get me back to them. The ambrosia was all-encompassing. Wherever I would go, it would go as well. That is a devastating thought for anyone who knows what these symptoms are like. To feel the discomfort and feel no power to rid myself of it, I would want nothing more than to *escape* the prison that my body had become.

When I should have been enjoying my life in Odessa, and all that it had to offer, I could not. I could no more enjoy my life than enjoy the rough texture on a paper towel after I had run out of tissues. It seemed that fate had fallen onto me – and decided that before I could do anything else, I would have to suffer through itchy eyes and a sickly voice for a while. I would have to deal with the ambrosia, as so many others did, for some indeterminate time.

Anyone who knows me will tell you, though, that I would *not* take something like that lightly. I was not going to allow the ambrosia allergy to control my life. There was *no* way I was going to stand by and let these symptoms control my life. If there was anything that I could do to change the course that the allergy had taken, I was going to find it. I was going to conquer these symptoms and reclaim my peace and comfort.

It has been a lengthy journey, to reach these goals and to meet these needs, but it has been worth it. My friends, you may be wondering if you have simply cared too much about the symptoms. Allow me to reassure you, however, that the effort this is going to take *is* worthwhile. The time that you spend ridding yourself of your ambrosia allergy symptoms will be some of the wisest that you have ever spent.

My questioning and my goals have led me to try a variety of solutions. I believe in the value of comprehensive research, after all. While others might have felt content to go with whatever solution they came across first, I was not. I wanted to know all the different things that other people had tried. It was important to me, even if I was not going to make myself a guinea pig, to be aware of all the different options. Every possibility seemed like a valuable avenue for me to explore, if only intellectually and theoretically.

The first option that many people consider is, it may surprise you to hear, *moving*. They will uproot their whole lives to get away from ambrosia, finding new careers and even immigrating to other countries.

It is frustrating to realize that people would give up their homes because of this pest. That is the reality of ambrosia, though. It is such a burden on people that they will leave behind everything they know to leave it in their past. After all of the work that they have done, they will forego the sense of permanence that is their *right*, for some air a little less ridden with the ambrosia particles.

Of course, I adore Odessa. Leaving was never an option for me. Whatever *else* it took, I was up for it. There was no way I could have even entertained the notion of leaving behind this city. Here, I have made a life for myself. I have built a business, fallen in love with a one-of-a-kind woman, and started a family. While I have made friends all around the world, some of my closest connections are in Odessa. The way that I saw it, if leaving Odessa or living with ambrosia were my only options, then I would choose to live with ambrosia.

That is why I searched as passionately as I did. There was no other way for me. I *had* to cure my allergy, and while I was doing so, I had to remain in the city that I cherished. That added an extra difficulty to my challenge. Those who were able to pick up their lives and move never had to think about ambrosia *like this*. They never had to think about their allergy and themselves as *cohabitants*, sharing a city, sharing a home.

My wife, who is a doctor, provided some valuable counsel

to me. Because she is such a firm believer in natural treatments and minimal interventions, she guided me toward supplements. She and I agreed that whatever solution I chose, it should *not* feel like more of an imposition than the symptoms themselves. Antibiotics and other hard medications were off the table for us. It was simply unacceptable to think that to solve a natural-world problem, we would have to get something that chemists had cooked up in a lab. For this problem at least, we were confident that we could find something more gentle and nourishing.

My family doctor agreed. She told me that she preferred natural sources. Treating me well, she pointed me toward vitamins and herbs that would help solve my problem. If I drank a little bit of herbal tea every day, then that would strengthen my system so that the ambrosia allergy symptoms never seemed as harsh. Combined with some physical activities, like light exercises and stretches, it would fortify me against the particles that had wreaked such havoc on my life.

There is no way for me to overstate what a difference this combination of steps has made for me. Simple vitamins, simple exercises: those were all that it took for me. Because of my natural efforts, I have taken my life *back* from the ambrosia. Every day is a gift, once again. Each breath is calming and soothing, the way that it ought to be. I no longer fear the sleepless nights or the wearying days. My body is running at capacity, and because it is, I am happy and relaxed.

Today, my life is *not* ambrosia-free. Ambrosia is a reality for all of us who live in Odessa. Yet, I have found a way to coexist with it. It is a pest that bothers me no more.

This book is a tool for all Ukrainians, but especially for the people of Odessa, those suffering as I have. You can take *your* life back, if ambrosia has stolen it.

Here's how.

CHAPTER 3

WHAT YOU CAN DO

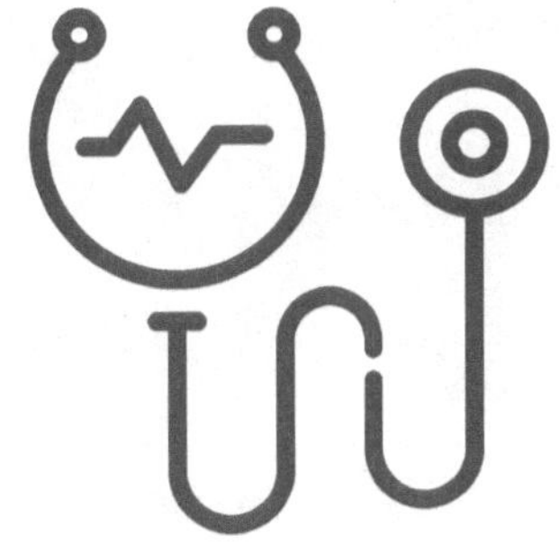

More than a quarter of all the people in Odessa are suffering from ambrosia today. That is a huge number no matter how you look at it. In a city of approximately a million, that means more than 250,000 people are dealing with the symptoms that I have described for you. Forget about the flu, and forget about the cold. At times when people should be healthy and enjoying their lives, they instead are dealing with the constant burden of ambrosia allergens. They feel trapped, and with plenty of reason. To date, no one has explained to them what steps they can take to protect themselves or manage their symptoms.

The history of ambrosia in Ukraine is informative. It started when someone brought it over on a vessel. After that, there was no turning back. Ambrosia, which is a pest, took root all across our fields. It then dispersed throughout our air, the way that it does in order to reproduce and propagate itself. It was an accident, and we are living with it today. No one had to target us with it. There was no need for anyone to drop it over our shores. Rather, it *found* a way. There was a vessel to carry it, a place for it to plant itself, and that was it.

Like any other pest, it appeared slowly in most places. Few people would have noticed the allergens in the early days. Only the hyper-sensitive would have seen a doctor or reported their symptoms, as anything more than a casual tickle in the throat. Little by little, it became more extreme. It ingrained itself in our lives. We were left without any recourse, without any defense. The ambrosia was more effective than any other invasion could be, all because it happened invisible to the naked eye. No one could point it out in the air or catch it with a net.

Today, the ambrosia plants are *everywhere*. This is the moment to which all of that history has led. We are dealing with the effects of an enemy that has embedded itself into our society. There is nothing we can do to change any of that, unfortunately. Nothing that we say, none of the choices that we make,can rid us of the ambrosia. What we *can* do is understand the pest. We can recognize how it functions and why it is so capable of hurting our quality of life. By doing so, we can move forward.

We can *conquer* it, the same way that it has hurt us - from within.

The problem is the worst for three months of the year. Those three months, we are most vulnerable to it. The symptoms become more noticeable. Some people who have gotten used to some morning congestion will experience fully formed allergic reactions. Their throats may feel so congested that they can hardly breathe at all. Each breath they *do* manage to take will become painful. As they lose sleep, they will take it out on the people around them. They will create conflict where there ought to be harmony.

As we get into September, we need to fill ourselves with vitamins. It is difficult to go overboard in this area. Whatever vitamins you feel are deficient in your body, those are the ones that you need to take *more*. You may consider getting an at-home vitamin test or even getting your blood tested with a professional, to pinpoint your greatest deficiencies. Analyze your health and the measures that you are already taking to protect your systems. Then, *act* on the knowledge and insights that you have gleaned from that information.

Whenever possible, get your vitamins from natural sources. Kiwi and strawberry are both delicious foods *packed* with vitamins. You may consider adding one or both of these fruits to your first meal, so that the vitamins can work their way through your digestive system and into your bloodstream as you get your start on the day. Other superfruits, like goji berries, are excellent additions to your daily diet. There are many ways to consume them, including protein shakes and energy bars. Pick something that you *enjoy* consuming so that it does not turn into one more chore that you need to do.

The ambrosia attacks while our immune systems are down. This means that if you are not taking care of your overall health, it is going to become much harder for you to maintain your normal state. You will feel the symptoms creeping up on you earlier in the year and then staying for longer. They may become more severe, even causing your health to degrade into illness as time goes on. Whatever your experience is, respond appropriately. Work out as much as possible, to keep your cardiovascular system strong and supportive of your immune systems.

It is also smart to get an expert opinion about your condition. I would like to suggest that anyone facing an ambrosia problem should visit the allergy center. See what the specialists there can tell you about your symptoms and about the advice that they have to offer. Because they are working with your neighbors, people who are dealing with the same allergen levels that you are, they will be able to provide suggestions that are specific to your location and your background.

Whatever else you do, my suggestion is to stick with natural solutions, as my doctor advised me. Stronger medications are appropriate during emergencies only. If you overuse them, you will become immune to them, putting you in a precarious situation when emergencies *do arise*.

ReO Water has also been very helpful for me. Drink one bottle per day. Put it in a spoon and stir it into a cup. This is a delicious, straightforward, and reliable method for adding support and leverage to your immune systems. They will become quicker and more powerful in their responses to the allergens that are making their way into your nasal passage and the rest of your body.

On top of that, you can avoid nasal drip by using Aqua Maris. This substance will clean your nostrils, in a manner that is much gentler than medical nose cleaners. By using Aqua Maris, you will abide by the "natural-first" principles that have worked for me.

Another strategy is to clean out your nose, to rid yourself

of toxins. The neti pot, which is popular worldwide for its simplicity and its efficacy, will run water (either distilled or salinated) through your nasal passage. It will then wash out the passage, to eliminate the allergens that are causing your symptoms. You will need to repeat this process regularly, but as you do, you may notice that your body is able to *handle* its allergen load more efficiently.

For watery and itchy eyes, try to use some eye drops, something for regular use. Helo Komed is a popular brand of Ayurvedic eye drops, beloved because it is much easier on the eyes than laboratory-synthesized brands are.

While you are following all these strategies, engage yourself as much as possible. Stay active, stay busy. Throughout the pandemic, I engaged myself by writing books and by helping seafarers, and in 2020, I did not feel any ambrosia at all. In 2021, I was less engaged, and I felt the ambrosia again. There is a pattern there: when I work on something important, it is as if my body *senses* that there is no time for ambrosia symptoms.

You will also do well to associate with positive people and remove yourself from negative people. A peaceful heart and mind *will* work to your benefit as you combat the symptoms of your ambrosia allergy. Toward that end, you should also meditate for 20-30 minutes every day, to clear your head of any thoughts that have been bothering you.

Following all of these steps, you should see some relief – which will be good for you *and* all of the people in your life.

CHAPTER 4

BETTER TOGETHER

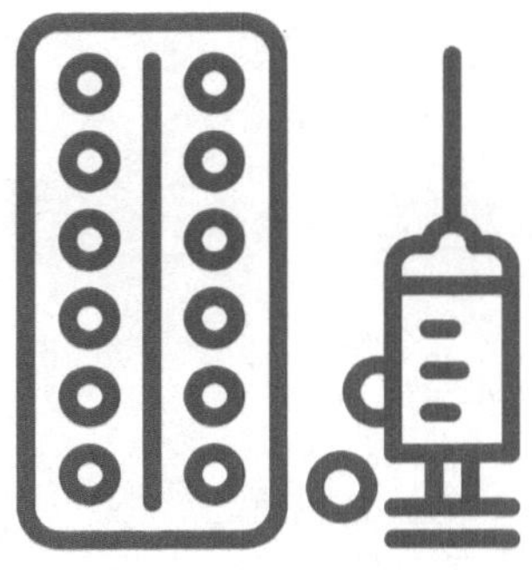

Do all of this and you *should* overcome ambrosia. Of course, our results will vary. One person may ingest tons and tons of vitamins, only to suffer from the same symptoms. Another person may wash out their nose one time and feel completely free of any ambrosia allergy. This is likely an ongoing process. You need to respond to your symptoms as they come up. When you feel some discomfort, or when it seems that you are getting worn down more easily, add something new into your routine. Tell yourself that you *will* beat your ambrosia allergy, however long it happens to take.

There is something else that I want to say, though: we need to unite together as a community to overcome ambrosia. While something like this is impacting our sleep schedules, it is also impacting our *economic lives*. We are suffering because of our ambrosia allergies in more ways than we may be aware. Whatever effort we are putting into our own individual care, it is not enough. Until all people in Odessa and Ukraine are free from these symptoms, there is still work left for us to do.

I will, for one, not rest until we are *all* comfortable and happy again. Until we can feel content in our own skin once more, I will continue to spread the news that natural solutions *can* make a difference.

We also need to find some way to destroy this plant. As gargantuan a task as that may seem, we need to keep thinking about it. Ambrosia has been attacking this country for too long. If it has not affected you, then it has affected someone around you. Every sniffle you have heard and every watery eye you have seen, it could have been the ambrosia allergy ruining someone's day. To show that you care about others, you must step *up* as we strive to take down this pest.

We have to support our community, to fight against ambrosia. I suggest that we pool our efforts. We will hire people who can carry out our plans and wage war against ambrosia. Although for the moment my focus is on pushing back on individual symptoms, it is much more sustainable for us to get to the root cause of our problems. The symptoms would never become an issue at all, if we could eliminate ambrosia from our lives. Decimate the plant wherever it lives – and watch as people wake up feeling better rested and more energized a mere day later.

This is an initiative that I have thought through extensively.

I have agreed to pay on behalf of my SELFLESS FUND to help out with this fight. Because of the love that I have for Odessa and Ukraine, I will not rest until we have created a better future together. We must *win* our freedom from ambrosia allergies.

GMC will also act on behalf of this cause. I am turning this into an international effort, on behalf of all those outside Ukraine also suffering from ambrosia allergies. To the people of the world, I see you and I hear you. I know that you feel as strongly about this scourge as I do. We are *one* in this battle.

Think about it like this. If we don't control our health, it will become more destructive for us. The mildest ambrosia allergy symptoms today may become life-threatening tomorrow, and without any warning. Those who feel they can "get by" with their ambrosia allergies may succumb to another illness, and regret all the time they never spent mastering their health while there was still an opportunity to do so.

At this time, if possible, I suggest that people leave Odessa and go outside where there are fewer poisonous plants. In

July, August, and September, take a vacation outside of Odessa, to remind yourself how smooth and pain-free your breathing can be. When you get a peek at that comfort, let it become the motivation that you need to handle your allergy symptoms once and for all. Remind yourself that however mild your symptoms may be, you would be better off without any symptoms at all.

In time, we may be able to look back on the "ambrosia era" and wonder how we were ever so nonchalant about it all. We may see the error in our ways – the silliness in allowing a pest to rule over us.

The thing is that it is not going to happen on its own. We need to talk openly and honestly about our situation, and begin to break ourselves out of it. You may want to pretend that *your* allergy symptoms are no bother at all. It is easy to ignore them until they become painful, after all. When your symptoms seem no worse than some light dehydration, you may convince yourself that you can pretend it is no discomfort whatsoever.

My advice to you would be to *act now*. Stop the pest in its tracks. See if a few lifestyle changes make an impact. If they do, then add in a few more. Keep changing your lifestyle, to manage your symptoms, until you have overcome them entirely.

As a bonus, you will become a healthier person overall. The vitamins and the exercise will do you a lot of good *besides* the smoother breathing and the clearer eyes. You will notice the effort that you have put into yourself. It will, in more ways than one, lead to *unprecedented happiness.*

Within a decade's time, I believe that we can all get there. We can put ambrosia behind us, sending it away from our beautiful land. Odessa is a strong city, where families raise their children to navigate any challenge. This challenge is no match for us, for the character of our homeland.

We *shall* prevail over ambrosia, one way or another.

ABOUT THE AUTHOR

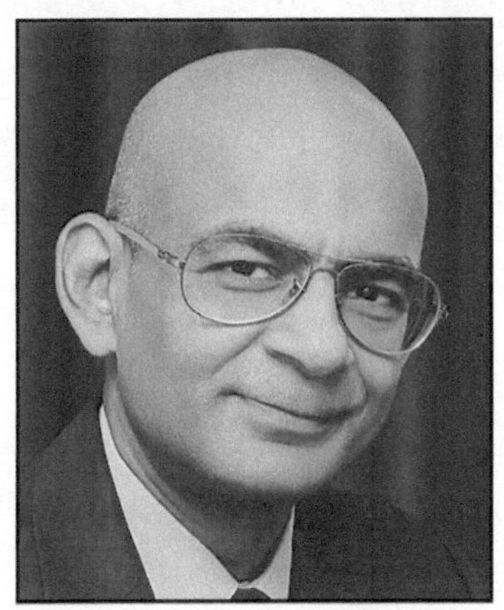

Dr Binay Kumar Singh, Founder & CEO of *Singh Marine Management Ltd.* in Odessa (Ukraine) and Founder & President of *Federation of Global Maritime Community*, is an entrepreneur, author, and public speaker. His life mission is to serve the world's communities and guide everyone through positivity, love, and enthusiasm. This is reflected in his simple and timeless life philosophy: "Treat people as you like to be treated."

Dr Singh has a Master of Science in Marine Navigation and a Doctorate of Philosophy. He is a globally recognized expert in international shipping with over two decades of experience. Dr Singh is also taking wonderful measures for the needy community of the society as well. His new project with the name "Selfless Fund" is specifically targeted to help those who are in need. Dr Singh has also launched his new company GSR which is going to bring innovations to the shipping and maritime industry. His efforts for the shipping industry as well as for the society is an example of his generosity and selflessness.

He enjoys pursuing multiple passions like singing, dancing, playing the piano and the accordion, and keeping healthy by practicing yoga and CrossFit.

Email: binay@drbinaysingh.com
Website: https://drbinaysingh.com

MORE BOOKS BY DR BINAY SINGH

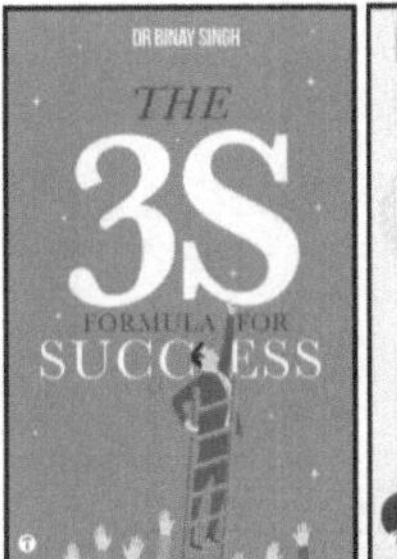

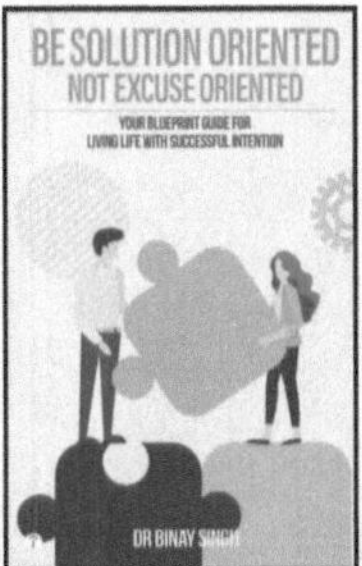

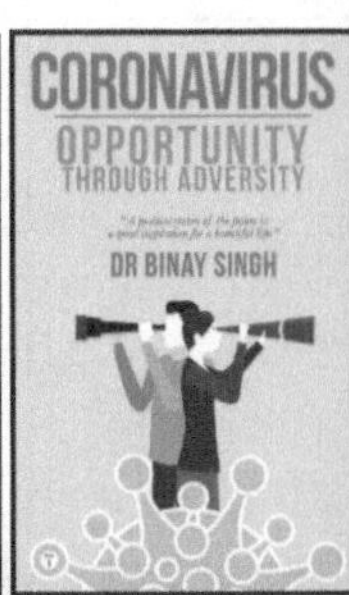

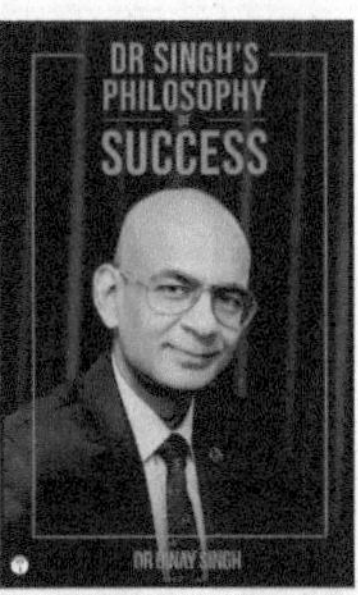

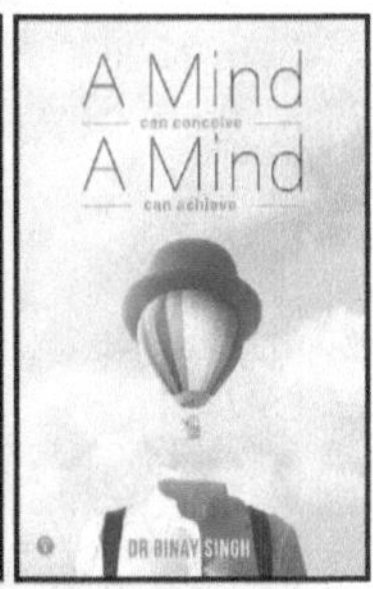

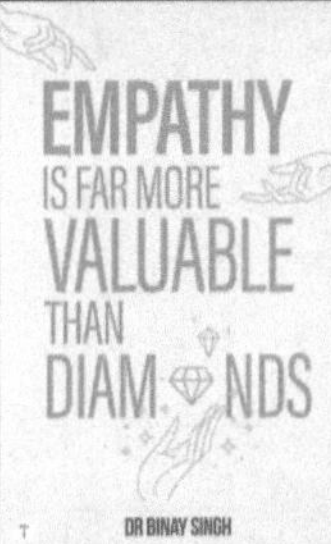

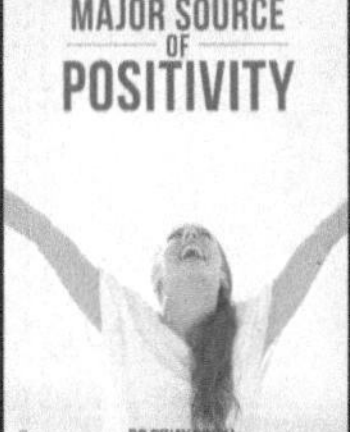

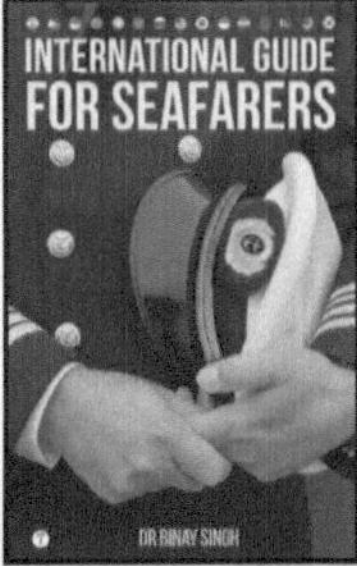

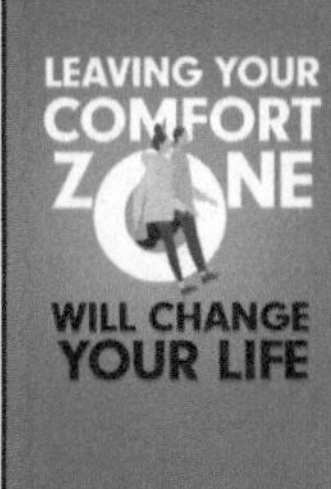

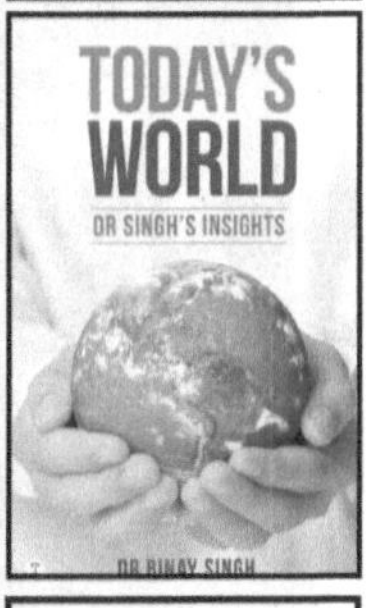

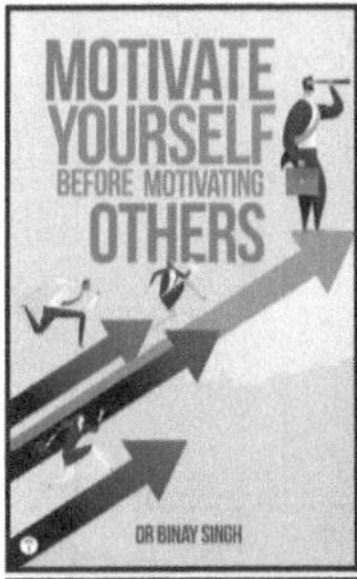

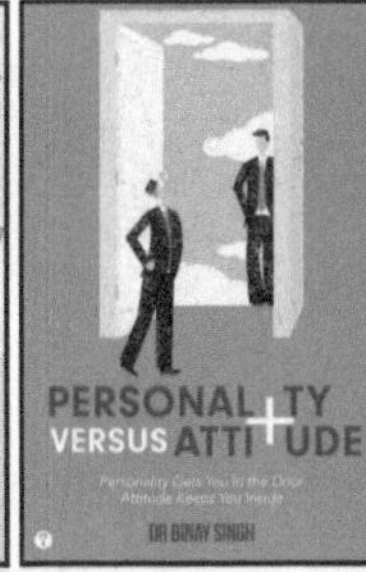

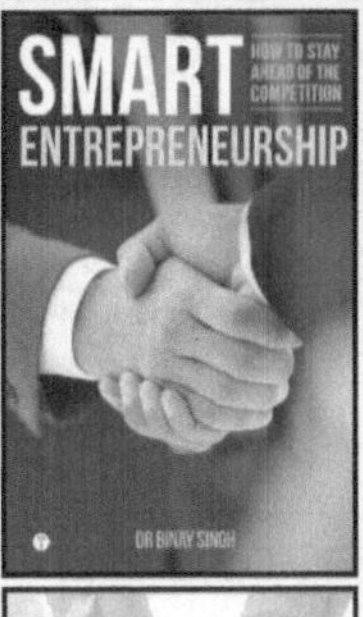

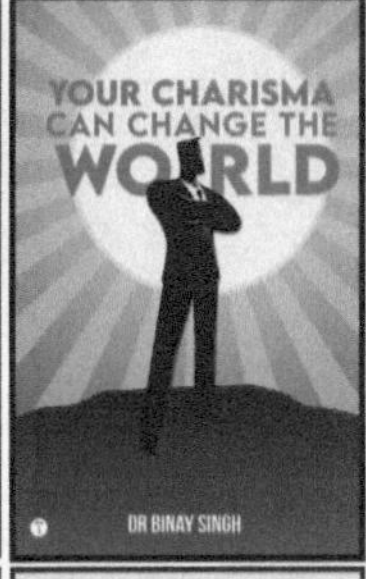

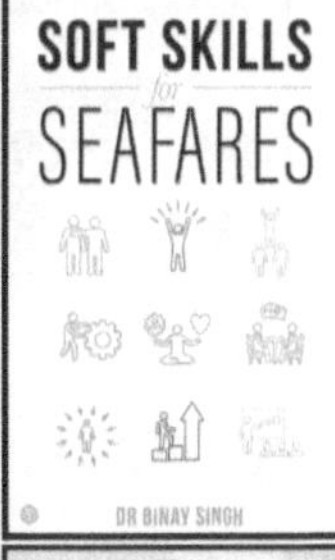

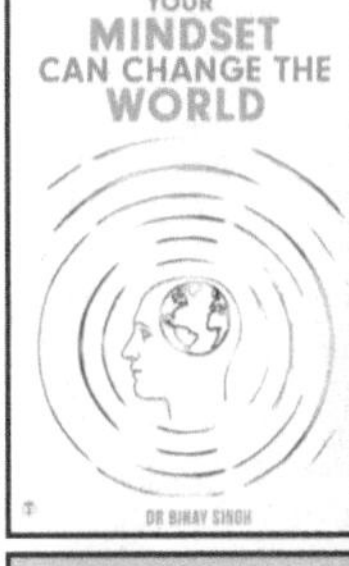

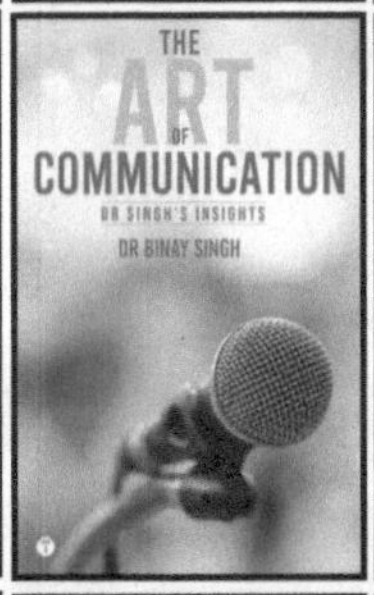

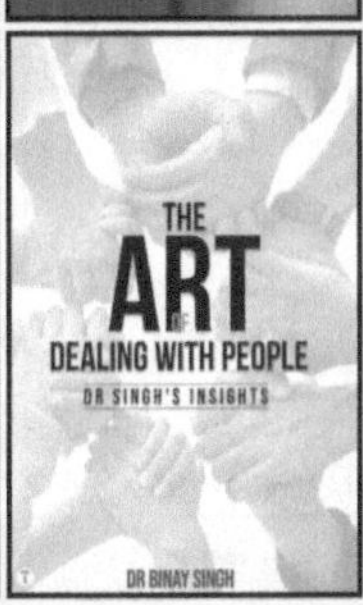

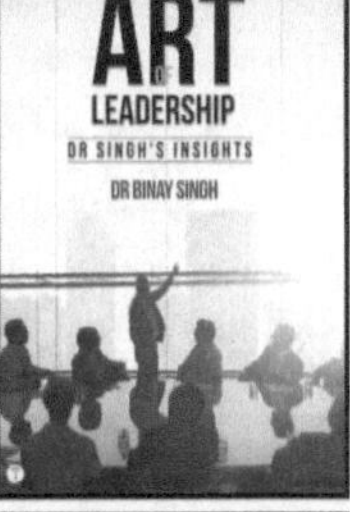

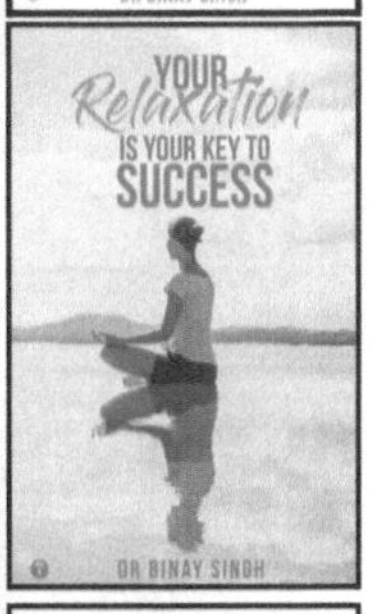

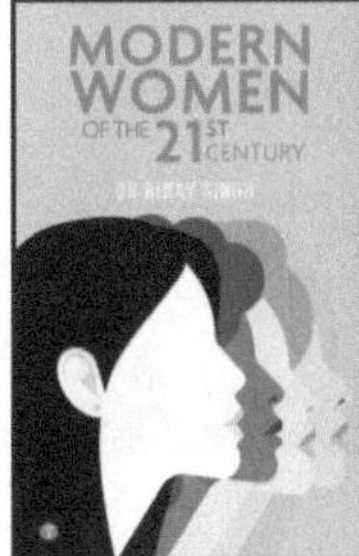

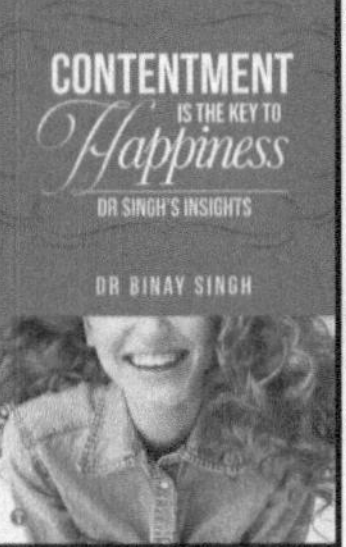

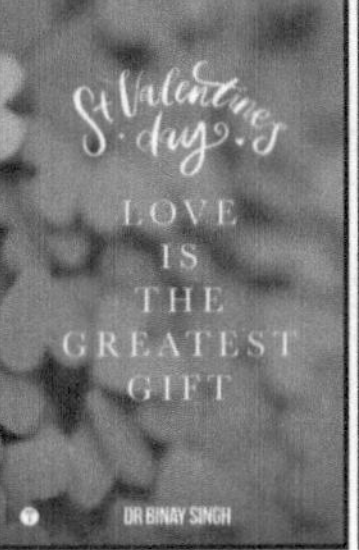

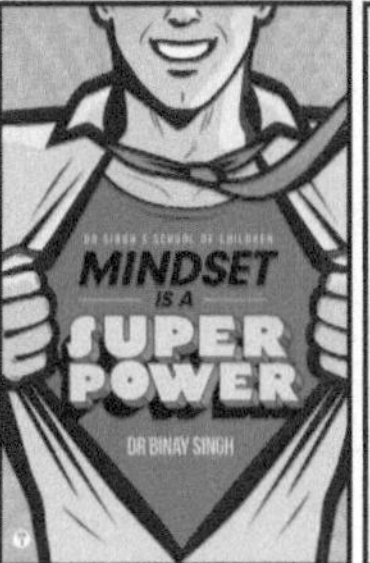

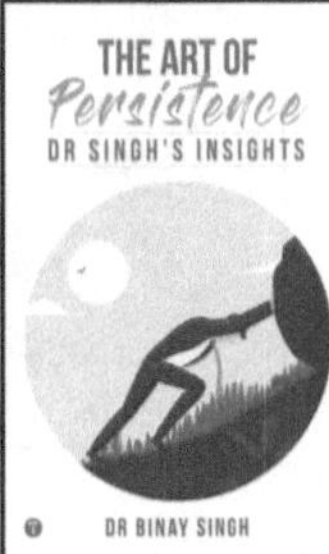

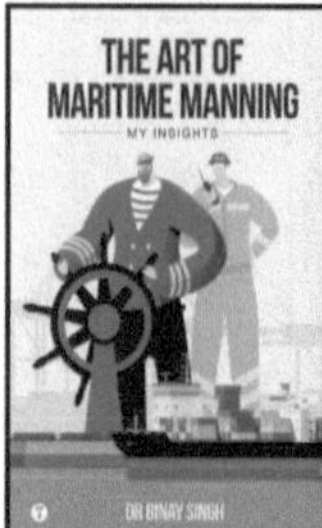
THE ART OF
MARITIME MANNING
MY INSIGHTS
DR BINAY SINGH

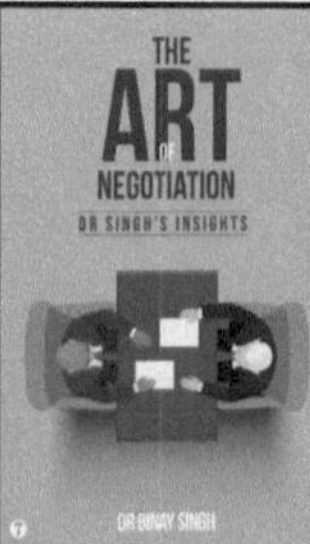
THE
ART
OF
NEGOTIATION
DR SINGH'S INSIGHTS
DR BINAY SINGH

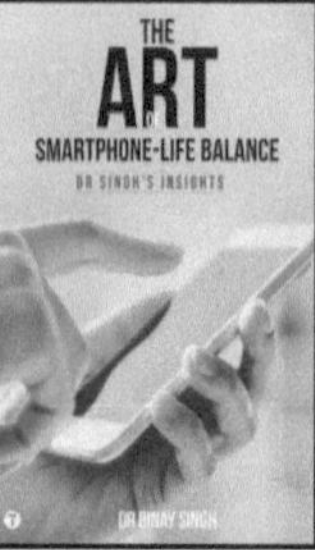
THE
ART
OF
SMARTPHONE-LIFE BALANCE
DR SINGH'S INSIGHTS
DR BINAY SINGH

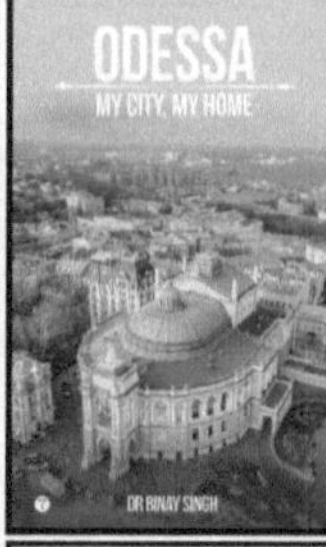
ODESSA
MY CITY, MY HOME
DR BINAY SINGH

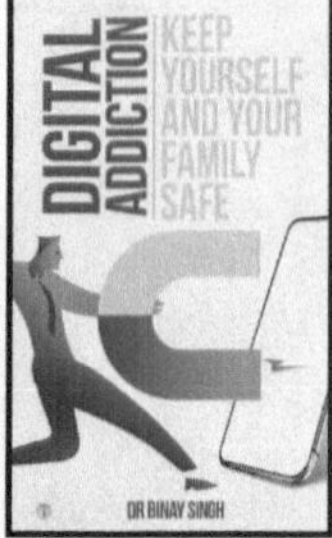
DIGITAL ADDICTION
KEEP YOURSELF AND YOUR FAMILY SAFE
DR BINAY SINGH

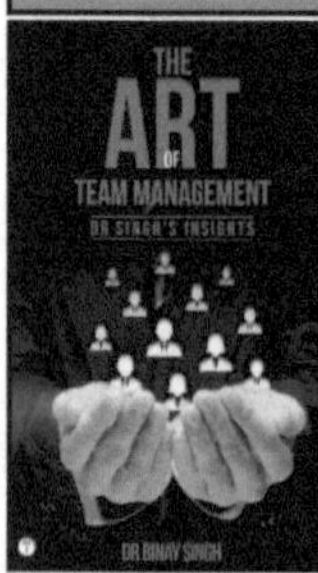
THE
ART
OF
TEAM MANAGEMENT
DR SINGH'S INSIGHTS
DR BINAY SINGH

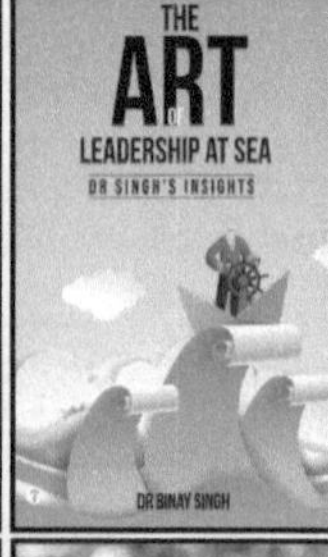
THE
ART
OF
LEADERSHIP AT SEA
DR SINGH'S INSIGHTS
DR BINAY SINGH

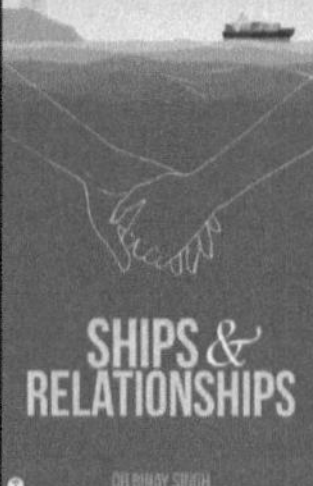
SHIPS &
RELATIONSHIPS
DR BINAY SINGH

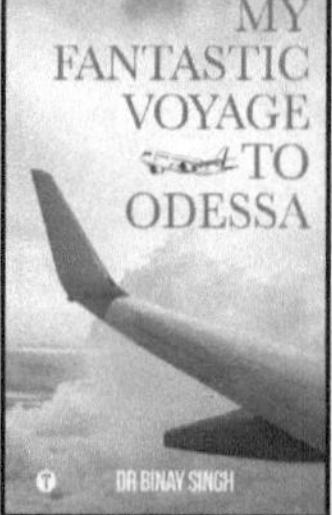
MY
FANTASTIC
VOYAGE
TO
ODESSA
DR BINAY SINGH

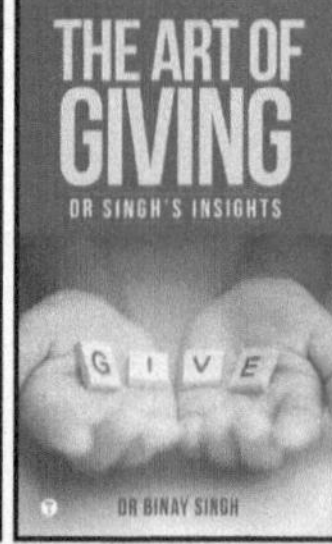
THE ART OF
GIVING
DR SINGH'S INSIGHTS
GIVE
DR BINAY SINGH

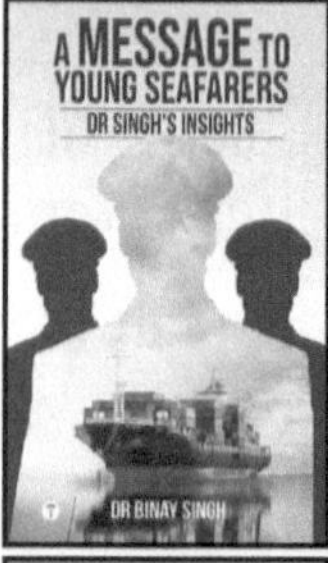
A MESSAGE TO
YOUNG SEAFARERS
DR SINGH'S INSIGHTS
DR BINAY SINGH

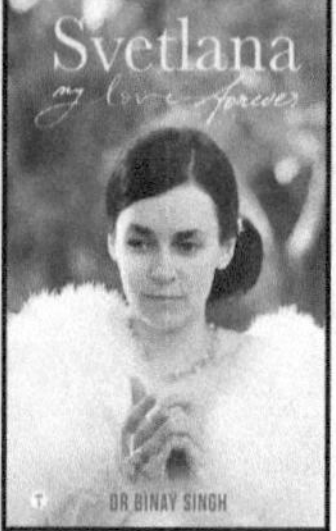
Svetlana
my love forever
DR BINAY SINGH

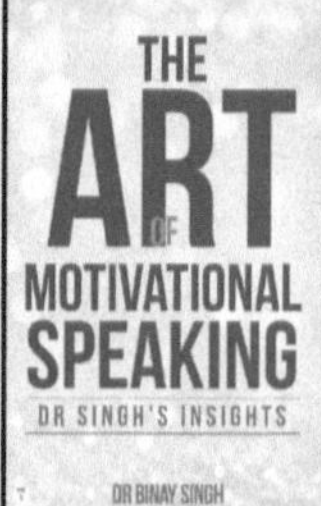
THE
ART
OF
MOTIVATIONAL
SPEAKING
DR SINGH'S INSIGHTS
DR BINAY SINGH

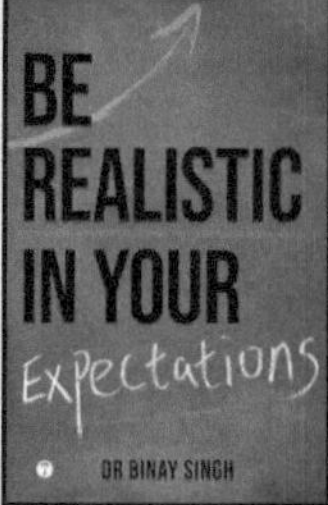
BE
REALISTIC
IN YOUR
Expectations
DR BINAY SINGH

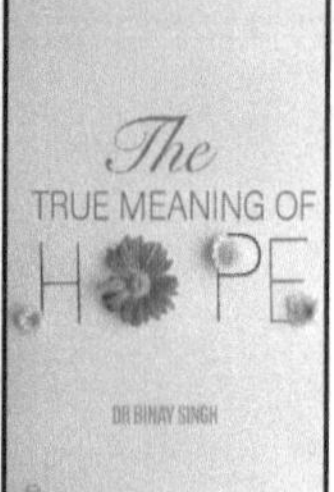
The
TRUE MEANING OF
HOPE
DR BINAY SINGH

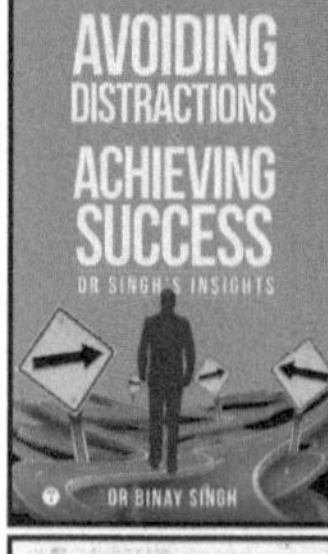
AVOIDING
DISTRACTIONS
ACHIEVING
SUCCESS
DR SINGH'S INSIGHTS
DR BINAY SINGH

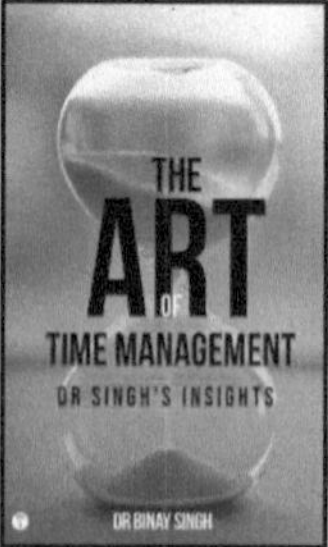
THE
ART
OF
TIME MANAGEMENT
DR SINGH'S INSIGHTS
DR BINAY SINGH

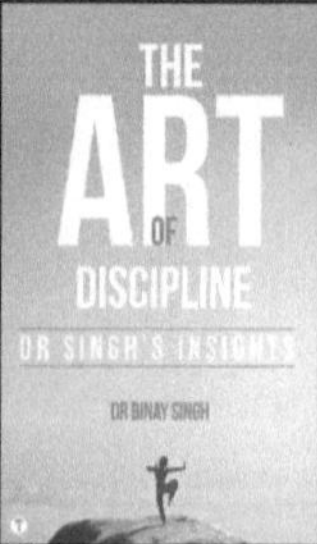
THE
ART
OF
DISCIPLINE
DR SINGH'S INSIGHTS
DR BINAY SINGH

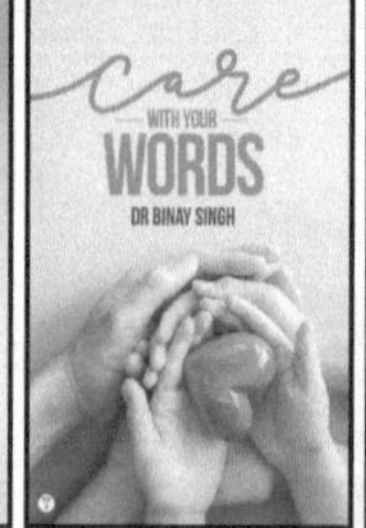
Care
WITH YOUR
WORDS
DR BINAY SINGH

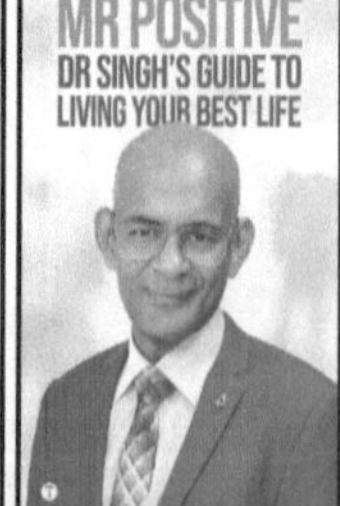
MR POSITIVE
DR SINGH'S GUIDE TO
LIVING YOUR BEST LIFE

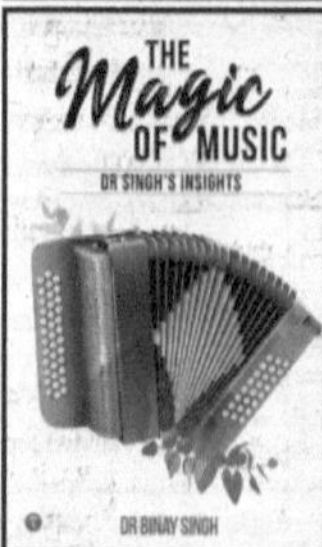
THE
Magic
OF MUSIC
DR SINGH'S INSIGHTS
DR BINAY SINGH

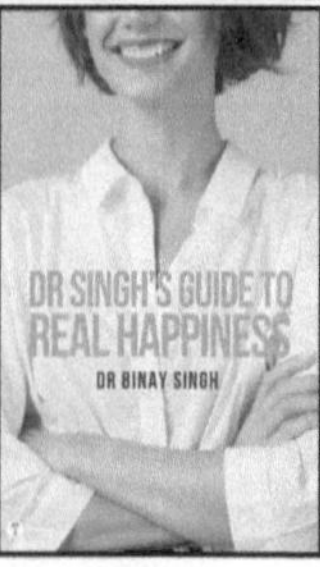
DR SINGH'S GUIDE TO
REAL HAPPINESS
DR BINAY SINGH

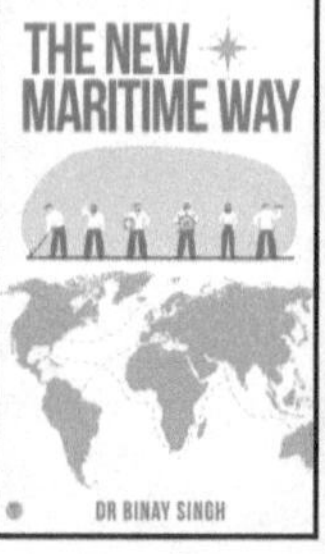
THE NEW
MARITIME WAY
DR BINAY SINGH

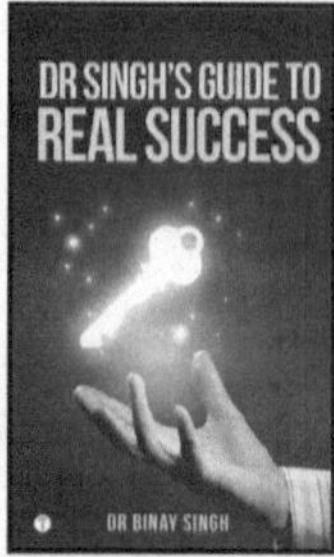
DR SINGH'S GUIDE TO
REAL SUCCESS
DR BINAY SINGH

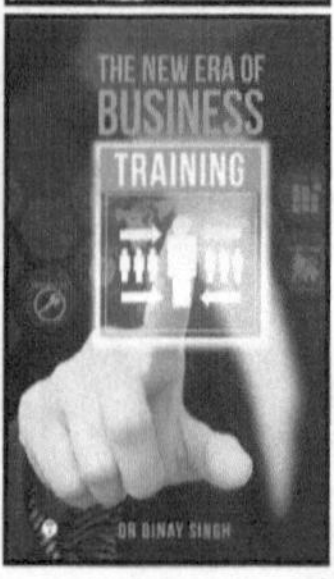
THE NEW ERA OF
BUSINESS
TRAINING
DR BINAY SINGH

www.ingramcontent.com/pod-product-compliance
Lightning Source LLC
LaVergne TN
LVHW041256150826
845673LV00008B/2618

* 9 7 8 9 3 9 2 8 4 9 3 2 9 *